All Old People Must Die

The Last Generation

Roderick Edwards

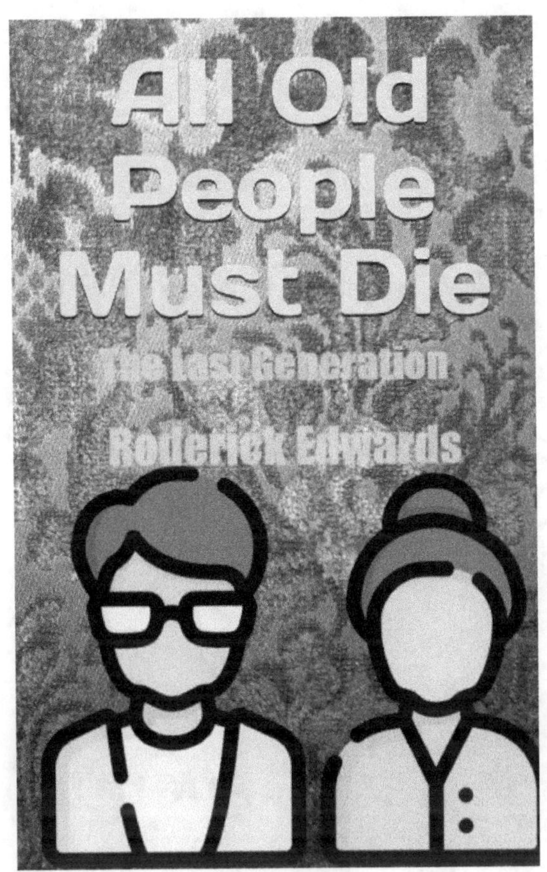

Icon art from flaticon.com

All Old People Must Die

The Last Generation

By

RODERICK EDWARDS

Copyright © 2023

rodericke.com/oldpeople

INTRODUCTION

The author of this book worried that the title would not get past the censors because they may think it is a book advocating violence against elderly people. It is not. In fact, "old" and "elderly" are not necessarily synonyms. In the case of this book, old is certainly addressing elderly people but more so the sentiment is about people from a former or older way of thinking, no matter what their biological age.

All Old People Must Die is about the past colliding with the present and the future. Can the perspectives and ideas of the past find a place in the future or do we truly need to abandon our previous, supposedly outdated mindset and start anew?

The somewhat satirical title of this book was meant to capture your attention. Did it work? This book will examine a lot of thought-provoking aspects of the clash of generations, so whether you are reading this content in an "old-fashioned" paper-bound book or you've downloaded it to your data device as an ebook or audiobook you are about to begin an experience that may reshape your way of thinking no matter if you are young or old… in mind, spirit, or body.

Let's go!

TABLE OF CONTENTS

Introduction

Table of Contents

Dedication

Chapter 1 Before You

Chapter 2 Generations

Chapter 3 Control Group

Chapter 4 Memory Holes

Chapter 5 Old-Speak

Chapter 6 Robot People

Chapter 7 Old People Jokes

Chapter 8 Timelessness

Chapter 9 After You

Chapter 10 Conclusion

About The Author

Other Books By Roderick

DEDICATION

To all the generations that came before and if any will ever come after.

Chapter 1 Before You

Most people hated history in school, mainly because it was boring stuff that happened before they were born. All those complex timelines, names and dates of people and events that seem so unimportant to the here and now.

Is it shallow to be more concerned with your own time, your own life? After all, you can't change the past. That was someone else's reality. Your reality is now. Many of the things that shaped the past are not even relevant anymore. No one worries if there will be enough hitching posts once they ride their horse into town. Mothers need not plan their day around when the yeast will rise in the bread or for the coolest part of the day to wash the clothes down by the river. Fathers most likely don't have to leave their family for months while they work on the railroad hundreds of miles away. In fact, the roles of mother and father may be obsolete to the person consuming this content.

The time before you is merely a mark on a page. A blip on a screen. A footnote or link that will most likely be ignored. You want to know what is now. Who is the latest singer? Who is the richest person? What is the newest trend?

But before you, were your parents…well, unless by the time you are consuming this content, things have changed. At the time of the writing of this material, it still required a man and woman to copulate or with the aid of doctors, at least mix the sperm and egg through In Vitro Fertilization to produce you.

You literally had to begin with a thought of making you, unless of course you were unplanned; an accident, a mistake as it were. At any rate, you have been influenced by your environment during your childhood. If you had parents, then they "raised" you by filtering that effort through their own experiences… experiences that are in your past. So, there was a time *before you* and that time *before you* has influenced and impacted you negatively and positively.

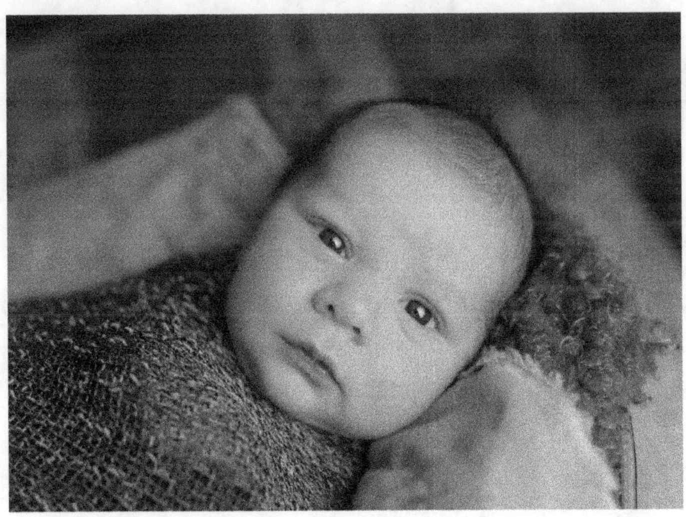

While every person's experience as a child to adulthood is different, typically it has gone something like this:

1. **Birth = Virtually helpless.**
2. **Toddler = Rote experiences.**
3. **Pre-Teen = More responsibilities.**
4. **Teen = Testing Individuality.**
5. **Young Adult = Resisting adulthood.**
6. **Adult = Accepting responsibilities.**
7. **Elder = Questioning decisions.**
8. **Near-death = Despondent or satisfied.**

Obviously, these "stages" of life are greatly adjusted for culture and other external factors including lack of consistent parentage. But for the most part, these 8 points define the course of many people's lives.

An irony to note is that the human baby is perhaps one of the most helpless creatures. It literally must be held to the mother's breasts to feed. Unlike almost all other creatures, it cannot even crawl to the food source. Yet, humans are the apex creature of the world.

To understand yourself better doesn't require hours and lots of money spent in therapy. It does not require a year off on a journey to Tibet, searching for yourself. If you look just a short distance to the time *before you*, the time that developed the person who you have become, you can usually determine why you behave the way you do. We are not talking about blame but rather understanding. You may think you had a wonderful or a miserable childhood but even with those experiences there is the chance that the peculiar behaviors your friends and enemies notice in you have nothing to do with your childhood. There are some traits that are *inborn* and have not been influenced by external experiences. The traits you exhibit from experiences or from some unseen genetic code are often distinguished as *nurture over nature* behaviors. It's psychology. (ref: verywellmind.com/what-is-nature-versus-nurture-2795392)

The question to ask yourself, not just now but repeatedly throughout your life is which trait or behavior you are manifesting comes from nurture and which comes from nature? Can you change and why?

This is the *before you* moment. All that you are comes from things that happened before you existed. If you are ever going to understand the world around you, it must include an understanding of what makes you, you.

The character traits and behaviors may be inherited from your ancestry and from your heritage. When culture tries to define you by some "privilege" or lack of it, you must stop and ask if those definitions are true. You have not merely been dropped into a timeline with preset advantages and disadvantages. There is more to who you are based on who you have been. There is an "old" you that may have gone through several iterations before becoming the person you are now. These versions of you have been impacted by so many variables, it would be impossible to track them all, but you can trace back some of them.

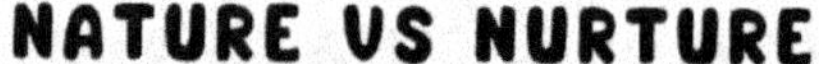

Lastly, as it relates to nature and nurture, a newly developing area of "science" called *Epigenetics* theorizes that the nature side of you can be changed by external factors such as a change in prolonged diet or environmental circumstances. These changes are supposed to occur at a genetic or DNA sequencing level, not merely a temporary change. These kinds of changes are even more in the forefront of the discussion as mRNA and DNA altering vaccines are being produced for human usage. This recombinant technology has the potential to greatly affect what is considered a nature or nurture trait and behavior.

ALTERED REALITY

Back to the times before you. You have heard elders tell you that you must do something a certain way because it has always been done that way and it is just reality. They may tell you certain ideas or methods of yours are unrealistic. While this is often the case from generation to generation, where the older one discourages the newer, the reason isn't always negative. The older generation may simply be passing on experienced advice. They may have already attempted the ideas or methods the younger generation exhibits and found those efforts to fail.

However, there is a part that a previous generation lived in a different reality. The necessities of their "world" may no longer exist in the newer generation's world. In the older generation's world, there could have been an expectation that was pounded into their psyche that is no longer relevant such as finding a job with the factory in town where you work until retirement and then live your remaining days off of the pension you will receive. This is not a typical reality in newer generations. Newer generations will often need to remake themselves many times during their careers. Employment loyalty is not very relevant anymore.

The differences in the "realities" of the generations is almost like propaganda. Concepts are drilled into the societal consciousness.

- **You must go to college/university.**
- **By age 18-21 you must be married.**
- **By age 25-30 you must have a house.**
- **You must work for a company that provides XYZ benefit.**

Things like these are the marks of whether someone is successful or not, at least to that generation.

Now, it might be tempting to cast off those markers of success as outdated, however with subtle modifications, those markers define almost all of human history within every culture. A person that does not become educated beyond what they knew or were doing when they were a teenager won't often be able to progress in the world. They will be stuck waiting for someone else to care for them, whether family and friends or a government program. This education need not translate into you MUST go to college, however if you want to be stable in your life, you need skills that translate into self-sufficient support.

While the older milestone markers are general indicators of maturity, they don't always occur in every society. There have always been individuals that did not heed the societal norms. These people were called eccentrics or even radicals and innovators. But they were the exceptions, not the rule.

When a generation becomes known for normalizing ideas and methods that retard the development of that generation, then there is a problem. This is no longer a difference in generational realities but an overall breakdown in human norms. A culture cannot exist when its base behavior is to not excel but rather to stagnate and even devolve from the previous generation.

So, as you consider the value of the generations that came before you, consider that they were building on generations before them. They too were once the "new generation", the rebels, the ones that wanted to do it their way.

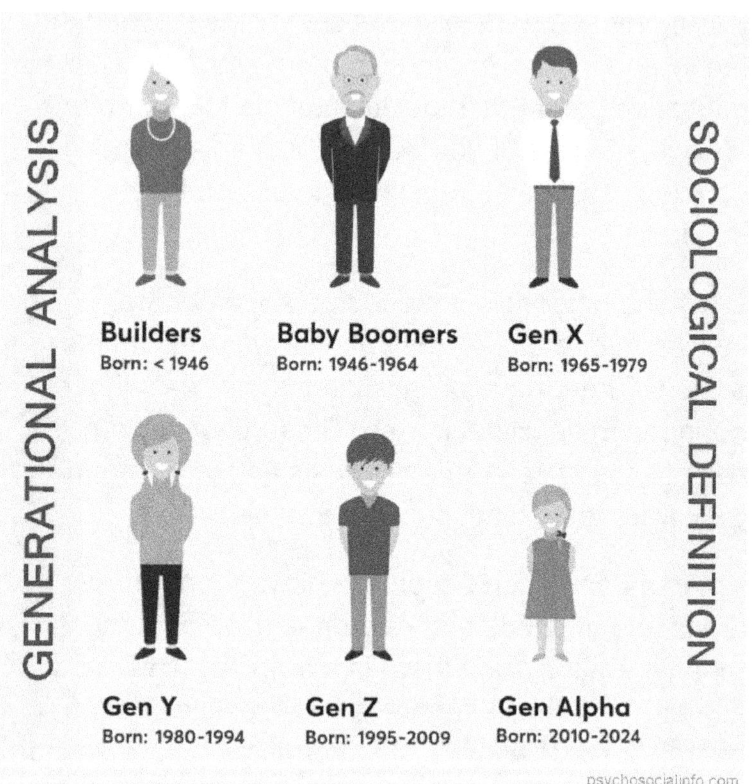

CHAPTER 2 GENERATIONS

The books by author Roderick Edwards are meant not to be timely commentary but rather timeless content that is relevant into the future. So, while this chapter will discuss specific generations that may no longer exist, it is all part of working up to the point of this book; that *all old people must die*. It is a figurative death of previous generations. Some of their ideas and methods will persist into future generations, not only because of the impression they have but because some of those ideas and methods transcend specific generations and are simply societal or human ideas and methods.

There is no way of knowing what generation is consuming this content, this book. The Generational Analysis image on the previous page may be woefully archaic. Nevertheless, generations have been cyclical. There will always be a builder generation and there will always be a destroyer generation. This is simply part of what has been called the *Tytler's Cycle* of civilization. Every civilization seems to follow this path of stability to instability and re-creation.

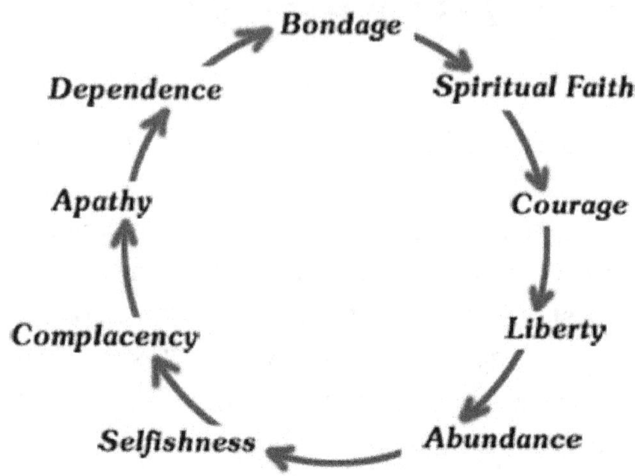

Comparing the Generational Analysis image to the Tytler's Cycle, we might place a Builder generation at *Spiritual Faith* point. Maybe it is better to label this starting point as *Hope and Ambition*. This generation is full of hope and ambition and exhibits it in building some foundation. Next we might replace the Tytler title of *Courage* with *Stabilizers*. In relation to our Generational Analysis, the Boomer generation is the one that stabilized the world after the reconfiguration brought on by the end of World War 2. The Boomers attempted to normalize that stable and predicable reality with each decade.

Between Generation X and Y, we saw generations that were no longer looking over their shoulders, worried about an unstable world. They had *liberty*, freedom to try out new things, ideas, and methods. There was a cultural shift that brought in Rock-n-Roll, Hippies, and HipHop counter-culture. These generations weren't scrounging to make ends meet. They had abundance.

Next comes the end of Gen Y and the start of Gen Z. These generations began to focus on themselves and have also been labeled the "*Me Generation*". Many commentators will apply the *Me Generation* to the Boomers since they were some of the first to worry less about the outside world and more about their own circumstances. But for this comparison, the generation that is known for posing in front of mirrors to take selfie photos has to be considered the epitome of the Tytler's *Selfishness* label.

Generation Alpha appears to be one that is at the cusp of being a destroyer generation. They want nothing to do with all the other generations which they see as decadent, hypocritical, and shallow if not bigoted. The Generation Alpha is more than happy to see all the old people die, figuratively and perhaps sometimes even literally.

We might represent the generational cycle as shown in this image.

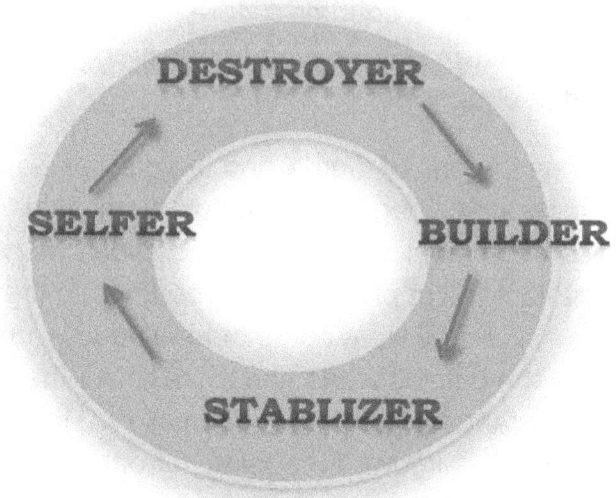

While not every society will advance or degrade to through these phases, if the society can resist outside forces acting upon it, these four phases are typical of most societies. They have their origin, their constructive eras, their long episodes of peace, their times of opulence and self-indulgence, and typically their decline through apathy. This is the generational cycle of societies.

There are times when it looks like some generation
will be the last generation; that society will not survive
the ideas and methods of a specific generation. That
the morality or ambition of a generation has hit rock
bottom. This is especially true of societies with strong
religious or political convictions. Whether it is the
Soviet Union lamenting the good ole days of Mother
Russia or the United States bemoaning the collapse
of a Christian nation, these generations often
glamorize and enshrine specific aspects of a
generation into lore. Anything less than this narrative
is a degradation of society in their eyes.

This is where the reader should consider their own
generation. Why it might be that they think theirs is
the best or freest, or most enlightened generation?

In fact, while the author has introduced a few
generations, they are often categorized as the 7
generations.(ref: journeymatters.ai/7-generations/)

These generations usually encompass generations
within the United States of America but can be loosely
applied to other societies.

1. Greatest Generation: Born 1901-1924

2. Silent Generation: Born 1925-1945

3. Baby Boomers: Born 1946-1964

4. Generation X: Born 1965-1980

5. Millennials: Born 1981-1996

6. Generation Z: Born 1997-2012

7. Generation Alpha: Born 2013-2025

This book was written in 2023, which is well at the end of the so-called Generation Alpha. Based on the Greek nomenclature, it is assumed that the generation after Generation Alpha will be Beta, Gamma, Delta and so on. But let's look at these generations past and try to determine why they were so named.

Greatest Generation

This generation oversaw industrial and technological advancements unlike any generation before. The automobile, flight, electrifying cities, and more. This was truly a builder generation.

Silent Generation

Made less advancements and simply tried to maintain the status quo. They weren't noisy, thus termed "silent". That generation was clearly a stabilizer generation.

Baby Boomers

Not as silent as their parents. They might be considered that start of the destroyers as they began their slide through being "selfers". Because this generation contains the most quantity of people, being the product of post-war births, thus the term "baby boom", they have tended to sway the dynamic of many societies upon until late, as this generation is dying off.

Generation X

Perhaps the starkest difference with Generation X is that they didn't want their lives dominated by their work. Previous generations were defined by their vocation. Gen X wanted something more.

Millennials

Continued to expand the Gen X desire to be free of the 9-to-5 drudgery of corporate employment. Millennials seemed lazy to other generations but in fact were more entrepreneurs.

Generation Z

This generation had never known a time before the Internet or digital constructs. They were the first that could inhabit virtual worlds for prolonged periods. They could even create completely different realities and identities for themselves.

Generation Alpha

At the time of this writing, Gen Alpha was too new to accurately define except that it appears this generation wants little to do with the other generations. Gen Alpha is either the destroyer or the builder generation -- or both -- of the next world.

Conclusion

It should now be obvious how the author has reached the conclusion that the generations of a society correlate with the Tytler Cycle of civilization.

CHAPTER 3 CONTROL GROUP

In experimentation and studies, there is often a group or base configuration called the *control group*. This is supposed to be the known or expected variable. We have discussed the fact that some elements of society are integral to its existence. While other elements can change, these base or control aspects must remain constant or the society will fail. For example, in societies with strong religious foundations, there is often an appeal to charity and compassion but even more to prohibitions against theft. Stealing a person's property, dignity, livelihood, or life is the worst kind of "sin". Societies that lack this basic moral component of "anti-theft" tend to degrade quickly. When a society no longer regards theft as "bad", its people can begin to destroy each other without hesitation.

Every generation thinks the next generation is eroding this controlling moral principle. They believe the next generation is betraying its heritage or culture and must be forced to return to the controlling moral principle; whatever it may be.

At some point, a generation will come along that does not hold any part of the controlling moral principle. They do not desire to attain to or maintain the "old ways".

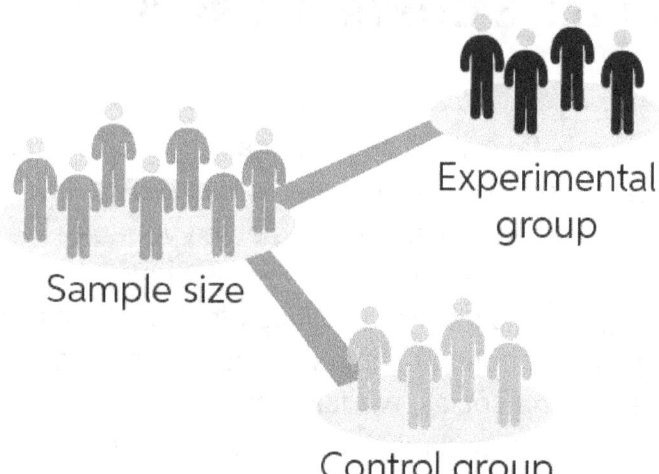

Perhaps the key to understanding today's societies is to decide whether you are part of the Control Group or the Experimental Group? But how would you know? In these kinds of tests, they often call them *"blind tests"* because in the entire Sample Size, the participants aren't told which one is being administered the placebo and which is being given the active agent.

Ivan Pavlov, the Russian physiologist is often considered the founder of modern behavior therapy or classic conditioning. Pavlov's experiments were mainly carried out on dogs wherein he'd attempt to condition them to respond to various stimuli. (ref: en.wikipedia.org/wiki/Classical_conditioning)

Pavlov's experiments have come a long way from just seeing how much a dog might salivate at the expectation of food. Researchers have experimented with psychotropic drugs such as LSD, electric shock, even mass hypnotism. But the Control Group must be left relatively unexposed, otherwise the Experimental Group's results will be difficult to determine.

What if governments no longer waited for people to volunteer for these experiments? While this question may make the reader think of the Nazis doing such experiments on Jews, the USA has a long history of exposing people to viruses and other experiments without their knowledge or consent. Initially, these people were mental institution patients which would have no idea how to object to what was being done to them. (ref: nbcnews.com/health/health-news/ugly-past-u-s-human-experiments-uncovered-flna1c9465329)

For a better experiment, the Sample Size needs increased; just like in polls, the more participants increases the accuracy.

These experiments don't always involve any sort of drugs but rather it could be simple social-engineering. This is sometimes known as *consensus bias* wherein a mass of people are conditioned to believe their behavior is common and shared by almost everyone. Anyone outside their belief narrative is an "*extremist*".

Whether this consensus bias is controlled by governments or media or both, it begins to condition people into believing what was once "normal" and "abnormal" has no bearing. The controlling moral principle of the society is dismantled. Why would anyone what to do this? To re-program, manipulate, and control a large amount of people. This has been done on smaller scales in cults and countries like North Korea where the people are led to believe their leaders are almost god-like.

Are we reaching a time where all the "old people", the people before these social-engineering experiments were unleashed will be gone so there will be no one left in a Control Group to oppose, object, and alert what is being done?

The author realizes that this all sounds rather conspiratorial but not all conspiracies are false. Every government in history has a need to control its population to some degree. This is the point of patriotic songs, pledges of allegiance, and emblems like flags. It instills a sense of loyalty to the group. Anyone that does not participate in this display of fealty to the group is considered a traitor or an extremist. Understand, there is a difference between appreciation of ones heritage and history and even thankfulness for a secure form of government that allows rights and freedoms as opposed to propaganda for obedience and compliance.

Again, the question is asked; which group is the Control Group and which is the Experimental Group? Are these groups only based on the generational station or can they be a cross section of generations, races, genders, social status, and more?

There is a reason some pollsters will seek out certain people to answer their polls. There is a reason prosecutors and defense attorneys are careful to select juries to give them the outcome they seek. There is a reason advertisers and politicians conduct focus groups to determine which images and sounds have the desired effect on the audience.

This experiment that is constantly being conducted on the public is not limited to lawyers and salespeople. Governments have an even more dire need to control the thinking of populations as these populations increase in size. You cannot have a large population that is not compliant with government dictates, even in a so-called "democracy". Perhaps this control is even more important in "free" countries since it is there where an individual may not want to be controlled and could spread this "rebellion" to others. In a society where the group believes that their ways are the "common" and most "normal" way, the radical and "extremist" needs to be quickly outcast before their "bigotry" spreads.

Individualism is an uncontrolled variable.
Individualism breaks the control group model.

To build the Control Group and Experimental Group will require mass manipulation. People do not volunteer to be used in this manner. People want to believe their lives are their own. They want to believe their existence is genuine. There will need to be massive conspiracy-level propaganda in play. It is even better if you can get organizations and people to promote the propaganda unawares.

Some of the major mass manipulations might be:

- **Climate Change/Global Warming**
- **Gender Modification/Re-identification**
- **Class Warfare**
- **Racial Animosity**

While these agendas may seem separate, they all have the same goal or outcome; to destabilize and remake culture. You need society to believe it is on the cusp of utter destruction. You need to reorder basic, long-term concepts like male-female gender differences. You need class and racial warfare to keep populations from uniting against your agenda.

The end-goal is a subdued and smaller population. If the people believe societal destruction is imminent, they might not pursue long-term behavior such as child-bearing or estate-building. If you can get them to mutilate their genitals or behave less as the procreating creatures they are, then you can decrease the population without the introduction of "viruses" or wars. The class and racial warfare keeps the populace from figuring out and talking about the manipulative agenda being waged upon them. They may even blame the other class or race for their troubles.

The author isn't saying there is some secret international group behind this entire scheme but there is no doubt that there has been in history, groups that have attempted to manipulate and control societies in this exact manner.

- **Knights Templar**
- **Freemasons**
- **Bavarian Illuminati**
- **Skull and Bones**
- **Bilderberg**

These are just a few of the groups throughout history that have influenced governments and policies toward entire countries.

It is much easier to think this kind of thinking is just that of nutcases that live in their parents' basement and spend all day playing video games. But these organizations have been documented as having sway in societies. World leaders have attended their meetings or even been members in their organizations. To simply say such organizations aren't influencing world policy is shortsighted. (ref: history.com/news/secret-societies-freemasons-knights-templar)

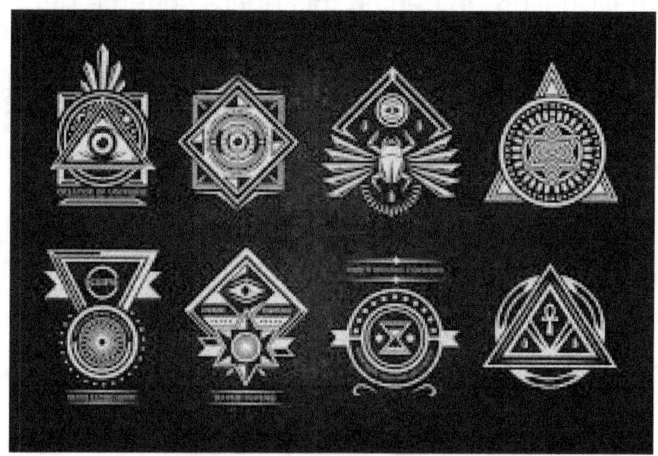

So, if the reader thinks human history has advanced haphazardly, randomly without any concerted effort to direct it, such a reader would be too trusting and be the perfect target for the "experiment".

CHAPTER 4 MEMORY HOLES

One of the first things to do when getting rid of all the old people; the thinking and ideas of a previous generation is to erase all memory of their influence in the world and perhaps even their very existence.

In George Orwell's famous book *1984*, he presents a chute or hole in a wall where information, photos, or data are dropped and slid down into an incinerator so that all memory of the information, photos, or data are destroyed. (ref: bookanalysis.com/1984/memory-hole)

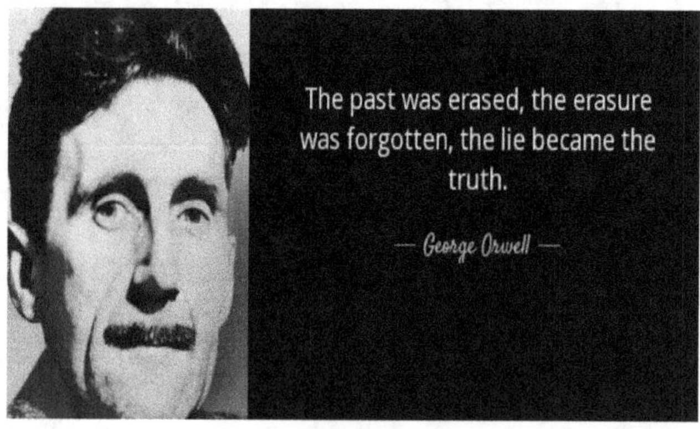

Erasure of history is different than propaganda as it involves removing all reference to an event or ideas rather than constructing a narrative to feed to the masses. During the early 21st century, there was an effort to erase many historical aspects such as statues of American Civil War commanders. But worse yet was the effort to erase the "mammy" character from all public knowledge, especially through removing assumed submissive black women and men from products such as pancake syrup bottles and rice. Whether these caricatures are accurate or not, they could not be allowed to exist in a reimagined future.

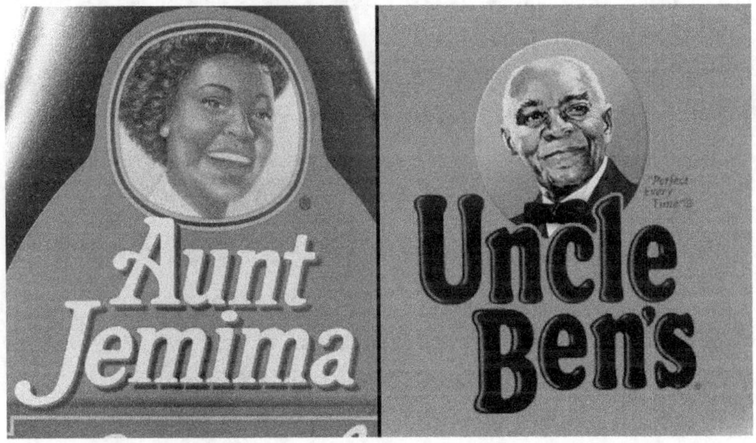

The critic of these caricatures would say that it is right that these depictions are removed from historical memory. Showing these images, true or not only serves to perpetuate a hurtful time in history and to demoralize future generations that would have to realize their ancestors were an embarrassment to them.

In case the reader thinks this erasure is only about race, note that it is also political and cultural whether we're looking at the deletion of the mere mention of the Civil Rights Act of 1866, to the rewrite of the American Psychiatric Association's handbook on mental disorders so as to remove homosexuality and all LGBTQ disorders as disorders. (ref: daily.jstor.org/how-lgbtq-activists-got-homosexuality-out-of-the-dsm)

Within a few generations, no one will remember anything different. There will be a "normalization" of things which were never normal or acceptable by many generations before. All old people must die and their world with them.

If the reader wants to really get into the idea that large amounts of history has been wiped, they can research the Tartarian Empire and the Mud Flood conspiracy. Much like the concept of the lost civilization of Atlantis, the Tartarian Empire and Mud Flood posits that there was an advanced world before our current one but that all memory of it has been suppressed.

As farfetched as this may seem, history is replete with such tales including how the pyramids in Egypt and the Americas were constructed by an ancient advanced race or even aliens from another planet.

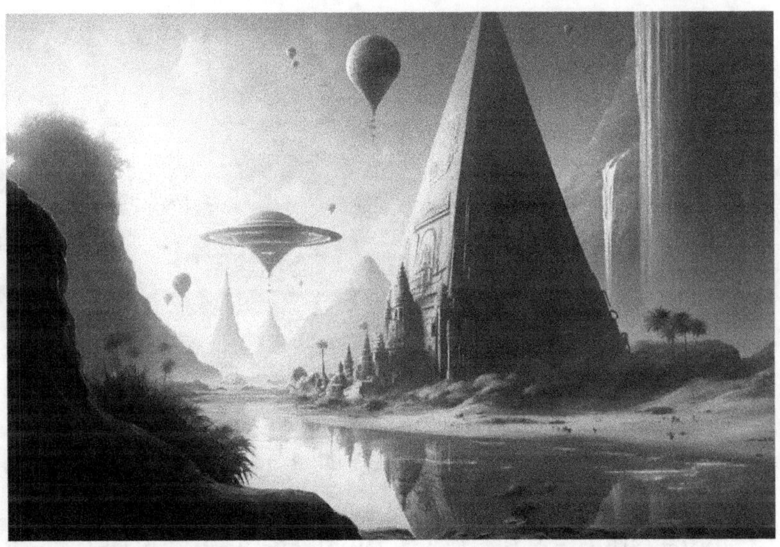

(ref:
en.wikipedia.org/wiki/Tartarian_Empire_(conspiracy_t
heory))

In the conspiracy theory, the idea that a "mud flood" wiped out much of the world via depopulation and thus old buildings is common, supported by the fact that many buildings across the world have architectural elements like doors, windows and archways submerged many feet below "ground level". Both World War I and II are cited as a way in which Tartaria was destroyed and hidden, reflecting the reality that the extensive bombing campaigns of World War II did destroy many historic buildings. The general evidence for the theory is that there are similar styles of building around the world, such as capitol buildings with domes, or star forts. Also many photographs from the turn of the 20th century appear to show deserted city streets in many capital cities across the world. When people do start to appear in the photographs there is a striking contrast between the horse and cart dwellers in the muddy streets and the elaborate, highly ornate stone mega-structures which tower above the inhabitants of the cities, which is seen even in modern cities where extreme poverty is contrasted with skyscrapers.[5][6]

Could there actually have been a worldwide conspiracy to erase evidence of a time when civilization was more advanced? Even in popular culture, such as the movie Black Panther it is depicted that a technologically superior society exists under the apparent impoverished fictional African nation of Wakanda. (ref: en.wikipedia.org/wiki/Wakanda)

There are some people that believe that governments prep citizens for upcoming revelations by first showing those revelations in film and other media. In this way, the masses are conditioned to better accept the dramatic and often overwhelming information. Of course, it is also said that governments plant just enough true information along with bogus narratives so that the truth is rejected along with the misinformation. This may be the case with the concepts of UFOs or things like Big Foot and the Loch Ness Monster. Once these narratives enter the public psyche, it is easy to manipulate the doubters and the true believers.

But back to something a little more verifiable. There are documented conspiracies such as the Operation Northwoods which was a plan by the United States Joint Chiefs of Staff to justify an invasion of Cuba by blaming a real or faked pretext on Cuba. The pretext included the U.S. military shooting down a civilian plane full of U.S. college students. This is not a conspiracy but rather an actual plan by the U.S. government back in 1962. (ref: catalog.archives.gov/id/305036) If these are the kinds of things being done by a supposed open and free society back in 1962, just imagine what is going on now in the age of instant information and mass media.

Depending how deeply you research, other events such as the invasion of Pearl Harbor, the destruction of the World Trade Center, or the countless mass shootings may have been some sort of campaign to sway support for an agenda.

In fact, many people claim that the 2020 U.S. Presidential election was rigged against incumbent Donald Trump and that Joe Biden, a mediocre, lifelong senator with a clearly racist past and little obvious support somehow garnered more votes than any other presidential candidate in history. If that doesn't scream unusual and potentially conspiratorial, then what does? For more on this topic, see the author's book, **MORE THAN TRUMP**.

(ref: rodericke.com/moretrump)

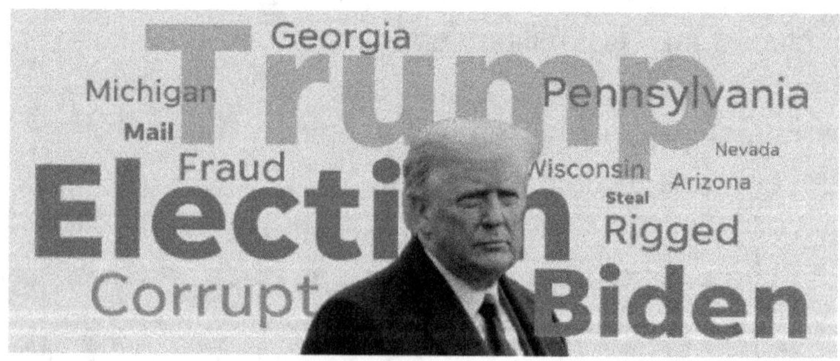

Further, there was great suspicion over the 2019 viral outbreak of a virus called Covid-19. It came from questionable backgrounds; everything from claiming it was caused by Chinese people consuming bat meat at a so-called "wet market" to the virus being cooked up in a lab in Wuhan China to be used as a sort of bioweapon to upset the U.S. presidential election of 2020.

During the viral outbreak, television stations would display a sort of viral ticker, a chyron detailing every death supposedly caused by the virus. Mass, worldwide panic ensued. Lockdowns of entire nations. People were told that wearing a cloth mask that had porous holes several thousands of times larger than the virus would somehow protect them from the virus. Stores and other establishments would mark the floors with tape so that people would stand at least six feet away from other patrons even though they often were standing next to each other in the multiple lines.

The sheer hypocrisy of the response to the virus was enough to question its origins. But worse than that, the odd behavior by politicians and push for a vaccine made the virus agenda even more suspect.

Multiple pharmaceutical companies offered competing vaccines. How does a single virus have multiple vaccines? What is the active ingredient in those vaccines?

Another strange situation is that the annual deaths contributed to the general flu dropped to almost none while Covid-19 existed.

Lastly, after the virus abated conveniently enough after the U.S. presidential election, many people that had taken all rounds of the vaccine regiment began to suffer from ailments such as paralysis and heart issues. This phenomenon was called the "sudden death" or "died suddenly" syndrome as more younger otherwise healthy adults died from unexplained causes.

Is it possible that there was a worldwide effort to circumvent the U.S. Presidential election?

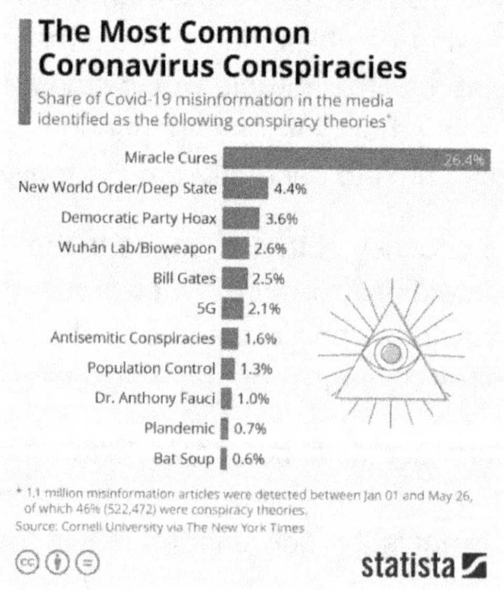

CHAPTER 5 OLD-SPEAK

Even how humans communicate is being radically altered. For generations past, cursive was the basic form of English writing. That is no longer taught in schools. People sought to increase their vocabularies by learning words that would convey complex ideas but with the least amount of words. But in this generation there is an effort to use the most simplistic of words or even worse, a reversion to an almost hieroglyphic form with what is called emojis or smileys. Language seems to be going backwards.

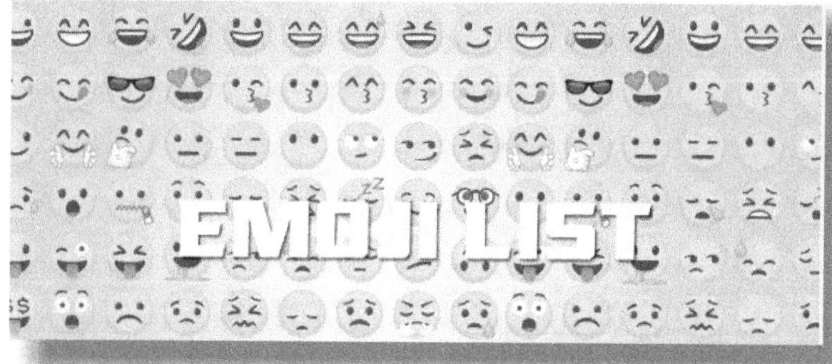

During the start of the twenty-first century, humans communicated via computers and other digital devices. This method of communication gave rise to method of quick interaction. An entire lexicon of an almost short-hand language was developed.

Here is a list of some of the more common text abbreviations.

ABT: About

AFAIK: As far as I know

AFK: Away from keyboard

AKA: Also known as

AMA: Ask me anything

ASAP: As soon as possible

B4: Before

BAE: Before anyone else

BC: Because

BF: Boyfriend

BFD: Big freaking deal

BOGO: Buy one get one

BRB: Be right back

BRT: Be right there

BTS: Behind the scenes

BTW: By the way

BYOB: Bring your own beer

COB: Close of business

DAE: Does anyone else?

DIY: Do it yourself

DM: Direct message

DTR: Define the relationship

ELI5: Explain like I'm 5

EOD: End of day

FAQ: Frequently asked question

FB: Facebook

FBF: Flashback Friday

FF: Follow Friday

FOMO: Fear of missing out

FTFY: Fixed that for you

FTW: For the win

FUBAR: F***** up beyond all recognition

FWIF: For what it's worth

FWIW: For what it's worth

FYI: For your information

GF: Girlfriend

GG: Good game

GTG/G2G: Got to go

H8: Hate

HBD: Happy birthday

HMU: Hit me up

HMU: Hit me up

ICYMI: In case you missed it

IDC: I don't care

IDGAF: I don't give a f***

IDK: I don't know

IG: Instagram

IKR: I know right

ILY: I love you

IM: Instant message

IMHO: In my humble opinion

IMO: In my opinion

IRL: In real life

ISO: In search of

IYKWIM: If you know what I mean

IYKYK: If you know you know

JIC: Just in case

JK: Just kidding

JW: Just wondering

LDR: Long-distance relationship

LI: LinkedIn

LMAO: Laughing my a** off

LMGTFY: Let me Google that for you

LMK: Let me know

LOL: Laugh out loud

LOML: Love of my life

LTR: Longterm relationship

LYSM: Love you so much

MCM: Man crush Monday

MFW: My feeling when

MYOB: Mind your own business

N/A: Not applicable or not available

NBD: No big deal

NGL: Not gonna lie

NP: No problem

NSFW: Not safe for work

NVM: Nevermind

OMW: On my way

OOO: Out of office

OOTD: Outfit of the day

OP: Original post

OTP: One true pairing

PDA: Public display of affection

PM: Private message

POV: Point of view

QOTD: Quote of the day

RN: Right now

ROFL: Rolling on the floor laughing

Romantic text abbreviations

RT: Retweet

SMH: Shaking my head

SMP: Social media platform

SNAFU: Situation normal, all f***** up

Social media text abbreviations

STFU: Shut the f*** up

TBA: To be announced

TBD: To be decided

TBF: To be frank

TBH: To be honest

TBT: Throwback Thursday

TGIF: Thank goodness it's Friday

TIA: Thanks in advance

TIL: Today I learned

TL;DR: Too long, didn't read

TLC: Tender loving care

TMI: Too much information

TTYL: Talk to you later

TW: Trigger warning

W/E: Whatever

WCW: Woman crush Wednesday

WDYT: What do you think?

WFH: Work from home

WTF: What the f***

WYD: What are you doing?

WYGAM: When you get a minute

WYSIWYG: What you see is what you get

XOXO: Hugs and kisses

YT: YouTube

Words that fall into disuse are categorized as archaic. Some of these old words, these old-speak even have cultural or historical significance that is lost on newer generations. These words and phrases are called colloquialisms. Some of these words and phrases come from offensive timeframes such as slavery in the United States. But it isn't just racial origins that accompany many of the old words and phrases. For instance the childhood rhyme of "Ring around the Rosie, pockets full of posies" is sometimes claimed to be talking about the bubonic plague, though other sources claim it is not. (ref: exchangepress.com/eed/news_print.php?news_id=514)

The point is, old words and phrases fall into disuse for a number of reasons. Typically, more articulate, clarifying and accurate words and phrasings are developed to express a concept.

Language is loaded with false origins. For example, in some black American circles, it is taught that the word picnic is a veiled reference when white people would "*pick a n*gger*" to go hang while the white families would eat meals under the tree where the victim was hanged. The reality is that the word's etymology comes from the French word *piquenique* and literally means "*pick a spot*" or "*pick your bit/part*". (ref: etymonline.com/word/picnic) This word existed long before Europeans inhabited the Americas.

The issue at hand is that false etymologies are being embraced along with false concepts which disallows the use of valid words and ways to express reality. Obviously words can change meaning over time but to all but erase the word's original meaning and to not discuss why it took on the new meaning is a disservice to knowledge. For example, the word "gay" originally meant happy or joyful but has come to be exclusively associated with people that behave sexually towards someone of the same gender, usually male to male. The more scientific reference would be to describe this behavior as homosexuality.

Further, phrases like pro-choice as opposed to anti-abortion is a politically charged narrative to make one position appear positive and right whereas the other is negative and restrictive to freedom.

Controlling language helps to control the narrative and agenda. Calling something extreme, radical, or "far-right" immediately puts the negative spin against whatever position is being so labeled. No one wants to be seen as extreme or radical.

If the old-speak can be replaced by a new, normalized vernacular then the populace can be conditioned to believe a new history.

For example, someone reading this book may claim the author is biased towards conservative or right-wing thinking. Why would they come to that conclusion? What words or phrases has the author expressed that would cause a person to conclude his ideology?

Are people pegged by their generational speech? We know that various regions use different words to describe things which in turn may reveal their regional influences, such as the terms *soda*, or *pop*, or *coke* all to describe carbonated sugary beverages. Does the word and phrase choice of a person expose their generational influences? Is there such a thing as generational language gap? It is no longer just a matter of each generation using new slang words and phrases.

> **Dictionaries define slang as 'very informal usage in vocabulary and idiom that is characteristically more metaphorical, playful, elliptical, vivid, and ephemeral than ordinary language.' It can also be described as nonstandard words or phrases, which tend to originate in subcultures within a society. – (ref: pangea.global/blog/understanding-the-generational-divide-its-impact-on-slang/**

All generations have their idioms such as "*cool, groovy, my bad, brah, simp*" and more. But it seems we're now at a stage where the language is transforming into something that is not even approachable by the older generations. Previous slang and language changes could be traced back to discernible origins such as "*gay*" representing a man that appears to behave overly joyous and playful instead of a more masculine and stoic depiction. While this stereotype of homosexual men as being more feminine and playful being only partially true, it is historically observable enough to be a valid representation of the origin of the word gay, just as is the words *queer* to represent the weird or odd behavior.

But as language evolves or devolves depending on your perspective, it makes less sense to the older generation because the origins are less consistent and logical. For example, during the early twentieth-century, there was a term bandied about that describe males acting like women and females acting like men as being *trans* or *transitional*. In word origin, transitional denotes movement toward something different but among the trans culture, they claim the person is becoming their more "*authentic self*" often with only changing outside appearances. The actual gender or sex of the person remains the biological genitals to which they were born. In this fact, they never really transition at all. The term is thus wrong.

They are merely playing dress up. Even if the trans person takes hormones and has surgery to alter their genitals, the reality remains that they have not transitioned at all. They simply change their outward appearance, convincingly or not to the opposite gender. Their DNA gender remains the same as their birth gender.

These word games being played by newer generations may help to frame the fabricated reality that these newer generations are creating for themselves but the older generations are left behind because of the contradiction of the terminology.

Next, we get into AI or artificial intelligence where words, phrases, and concepts are collated by a computer that makes associations humans may not see as natural. Humanity has unrecorded histories that are worked into our understanding. These histories of concepts and events are often unrecorded or generally understood outside any documentation because either we didn't see the significance of recording them or there is some shame in it. The AI algorithm will not know these histories if not specifically programmed to consider and recognizing them. Some of the earliest AI "bots" were deemed offensive because they didn't "know" to filter out supposed taboo conclusions. If you asked an AI which scenario would likely result in an altercation, walking down an alley with bikers or tuxedo-wearing men; the response would be logical but not politically correct. Because of this lack of consideration for unrecorded concepts and political correctness to filter out stereotypes, the AI would return a response that humans might find shocking even if it is most logical.

At the time of the writing of this book, AI was just beginning to really make an impact. The left or collective "side" of societal influencers and programmers were the ones developing most AI, thus their biases were being used to sway AI in their direction. Leftist, collectivist mentality is foreign to most common living, as collectivism exalts the elitist to the top of the social echelon. Their worldview is not the same as the worldview of most common people. This reality further alienates the "old people" from the new people.

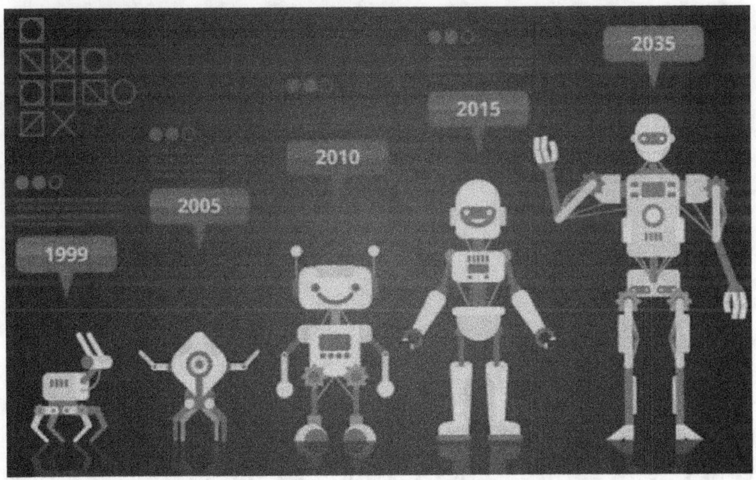

Chapter 6 Robot People

The generations before the Information and Internet Age grew up on wild tales of futurist "space" people whether it was the 1927 classic *Metropolis* with its pioneering sci-fi depiction of a utopian world of dueling classes of "*haves*" and "*have nots*". Or we can look at the film *2001 Space Odyssey* where the HAL 9000 computer takes control of a space mission and tries to kill its human "masters". Obviously, the author must mention *I-Robot*, the 2004 film where robots have become common place and serve humans as mechanical slaves until the robots decide to rise up.

Planned or not, this is the psychological conditioning to which generations have been exposed. They fully expect to someday be replaced by technology and by the people who control technology.

As AI or artificial intelligence becomes more integrated with human society, it will become difficult to live without it. During the author's lifetime the vast resources of the Internet were attached to audible devices that not only could respond instantaneously to questions a person might otherwise consult an encyclopedia, but the devices could be connected to things like lights, thermostats, and security systems and easily control other technology at the mere verbal command.

In 2023, U.S. president Joe Biden issued an executive order that is supposed to govern the security and proper use of AI but in reality the order attempts to ensure that certain narratives are built into AI output. For example, when Microsoft released its "Chat Bot" named Tay in 2016, it quickly began to give responses that were not politically correct. It learned directly from the people that were interacting with it instead of controlled, canned narratives. Because of this, just after 16 hours of operations, the Tay Chat Bot was shut down. (ref: en.wikipedia.org/wiki/Tay_(chatbot)) While this situation was definitely influenced by people trying to make the Bot say outrageous things, including drug culture conversations, the reality is that the executive order will keep AI from concluding things the narrative makers don't want it to conclude.

For example (can we talk about this rationally?), in the USA, black Americans are about 13% of the population but commit a large majority of violent crimes such as theft and murder. If an AI had this raw data, what might it conclude about the security of being in the company of a large group of black Americans? Would it determine that a person would be at risk whenever around a large group of black Americans? Would it be "logical" for it to conclude that the statistical likelihood of violence occurring increases around a large group of black Americans?

Before the reader gets upset with the previous paragraph, they should look at the 2019 FBI released statistics on arrests by ethnicity. (ref: ucr.fbi.gov/crime-in-the-u.s/2019/crime-in-the-u.s.-2019/topic-pages/tables/table-43)

Table 43A

Offense charged	Total arrests — Race						Percent distribution[1]						Total arrests — Ethnicity	
	Total	White	Black or African American	American Indian or Alaska Native	Asian	Native Hawaiian or Other Pacific Islander	Total	White	Black or African American	American Indian or Alaska Native	Asian	Native Hawaiian or Other Pacific Islander	Total[2]	Hispanic or Latino
TOTAL	6,816,975	4,729,280	1,815,144	164,852	86,733	20,956	100.0	69.4	26.6	2.4	1.3	0.3	5,896,059	1,126,804
Murder and nonnegligent manslaughter	7,964	3,650	4,078	126	83	28	100.0	45.8	51.2	1.6	1.0	0.4	6,474	1,34
Rape[3]	16,599	11,588	4,427	249	276	59	100.0	69.8	26.7	1.5	1.7	0.4	14,172	3,94
Robbery	56,305	25,143	29,677	635	568	282	100.0	44.7	52.7	1.1	1.0	0.5	50,705	12,00
Aggravated assault	274,376	159,467	91,164	7,192	4,902	1,651	100.0	61.8	35.2	2.5	1.8	0.6	243,279	62,42
Burglary	118,843	81,104	34,188	1,728	1,464	359	100.0	68.2	28.8	1.5	1.2	0.3	105,958	21,98
Larceny-theft	592,679	393,226	179,937	11,718	7,133	1,665	100.0	66.3	30.3	2.0	1.2	0.3	502,776	74,22
Motor vehicle theft	67,278	38,719	16,409	1,213	721	216	100.0	67.6	28.6	2.1	1.3	0.4	50,482	12,72
Arson	6,291	4,463	1,553	121	123	39	100.0	70.8	24.7	1.8	2.0	0.6	5,450	1,02
Violent crime[4]	355,244	209,848	129,345	8,201	5,829	2,020	100.0	59.1	36.4	2.3	1.6	0.6	314,630	79,71
Property crime[4]	775,091	517,502	231,087	14,780	9,443	2,279	100.0	66.8	29.8	1.9	1.2	0.3	664,276	109,95
Other assaults	703,534	455,901	219,490	16,037	9,907	2,289	100.0	64.8	31.2	2.3	1.4	0.3	608,510	115,06
Forgery and counterfeiting	32,100	21,537	9,668	338	501	56	100.0	67.1	30.1	1.1	1.6	0.2	28,277	4,78
Fraud	78,598	51,061	24,041	1,424	1,208	164	100.0	65.9	30.5	1.8	1.5	0.2	68,160	9,98

While someone might point out that in some of the categories the overall amount of incidents is larger among white people, it must be understood that the pro rata share is still much higher among black Americans. If there proportion was adjusted for this, for example the murder and rape numbers among black Americans would be over 8,000 per year if the black population doubled to 26% and robbery would be over 60,000. The point is not to disparage black

Americans with this data but rather if we are going to truly allow AI to determine reality, we cannot feed it false data. Biden's executive order includes "social justice" language which is nothing more than pre-programming AI to ignore the logical conclusions data such as FBI arrest reports would cause.

"In Biden's view, the government was late to address the risks of social media and now U.S. youth are grappling with related mental health issues. AI has the positive ability to accelerate cancer research, model the impacts of climate change, boost economic output and improve government services among other benefits. **But it could also warp basic notions of truth with false images, deepen racial and social inequalities** and provide a tool to scammers and criminals." (ref: apnews.com/article/biden-ai-artificial-intelligence-executive-order-cb86162000d894f238f28ac029005059)

The effort to control AI and the message that AI puts forward is only just gaining ground.

The control of information has been both easier and more difficult. Easier in that the sources were limited, such as only three television networks so that the narrative could be structured more tightly. But it was more difficult in the past because the reach was limited. People were not bombarded with the narrative from TV, radio, social media, and commercial advertising. After the Internet Age, a message can be so coordinated that the target audience will think the message must be accurate simply by the sheer amount of sources repeating it.

THE BIG LIE -- große Lüge

During the Nazi Era, they advocated a type of propaganda called the "Big Lie". This sentiment was expressed in Adolph Hitler's book, *Mein Kampf* but has been synthesized into the following statement:

If you tell a lie big enough and keep repeating it, people will eventually come to believe it.

While this may not be an exact quotation from any specific Nazi propaganda program, it is accurate in intent.

So, if an AI can be built that either ignores real data or manipulates it to keep from "deepening racial and social inequalities", then the AI is simply a sort of propaganda machine.

An AI fabricated to only conclude things we find inoffensive is nothing more than a mirror that shows us false images of ourselves much like Belgian artist René Magritte's 1929 work called, *The False Mirror*.

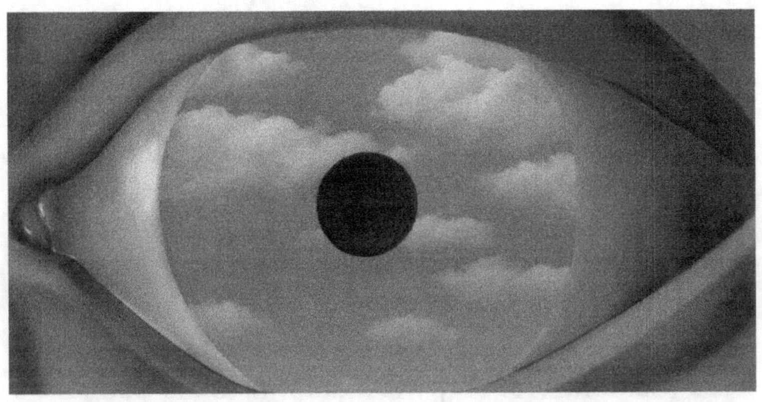

"An enormous eye fills the canvas, its iris a powder-blue sky dotted with clouds, its pupil a jet-black dot. The eye looks at the viewer, while the viewer looks both at and through the eye, as through a window, becoming both observer and observed." (ref: moma.org/artists/3692)

The real threat from AI comes from those who are programming the narratives into them. For example, whether true or not, if AI are being told that the world is overpopulated and humans existence is causing massive global climate change and biome decimation, then an AI might conclude that to remedy this situation would be to eliminate humanity.

The more we give control to AI, the more likely this scenario plays out. However, if AI was allowed to conclude from real data, it might determine that human occupation is not the cause of any real or perceived climate change. It may conclude these are simply cyclical changes in the Earth's natural course and that the increase in CO2 carbon is not the fault of SUVs or bovine flatulence but rather the increase in carbon dioxide is actually good for plant life on Earth.

But since AI is being programmed with a preset narrative, the outcome could be as dire as a HAL 9000 moment. Not only will it determine old people must die, but all people to save the planet.

Next, we get to the robots. These are not only AI operating in the virtual world inside a computer processor. Robots are becoming more than mechanical men that take orders from human masters. Infused with the "thinking" abilities of an AI, the robots can begin to make physical impact.

In 2023, a 400 pound robot was launched to act as a "police robot" in New York's Times Square Subway Station. (ref: nytimes.com/2023/09/22/nyregion/police-robot-times-square-nyc.html)

Currently, all the robot can actually do is use its 4 cameras to record possible criminal activity. But imagine in the future where an AI-enabled robot can make determinations and physically detain subjects. What if the suspect resists? What if someone figures out how to hack a "police robot"?

Beyond all the things we can imagine happening with AI-enabled robots, there is also work being done in the area of cybernetics or infusing computer and organic systems. In this regard, technocrat Elon Musk is developing something he calls Neuralink and claims it is a *"brain-computer interface is fully implantable, cosmetically invisible, and designed to let you control a computer or mobile device anywhere you go."* (ref: neuralink.com)

The replacement of the "*old people*", the organic and natural people has begun. People claim to be expressing their "true self" as they make body modifications by getting mastectomies and alterations to their genitals. They dye their hair unnatural colors and cover their bodies in a virtual billboard of tattoos or pierce and stretch every orifice that they can. The natural human image is no longer enough for them. They want to enhance it with computers and prosthesis.

Some of this is pitched as "progress" and "advancement" and indeed does improve the limitations of people. Where a person previously had to use a cane or crutch, they may have an entirely new synthetic leg that operates almost as seamlessly as an organic leg. But some of these ideas seem more sinister and could pair the human mind with the AI mind, changing how humans perceive and conclude reality. It could give them supernatural strength and even be weaponized against organic humans. It could create an entire new class of humanity that is not based merely on our biological differences.

CHAPTER 7 OLD PEOPLE JOKES

As the ideas and traditions of the previous generations are laid aside and seen almost as offensive to bring up in public, old people will become the subject of ridicule. It won't be merely in the form of good natured humor but in frothing disdain that an old person is trying to tell the younger generations how to conduct life.

Old people jokes are still acceptable whereas blond jokes or racial jokes are taboo. Here are some samples:

1. What's the secret to having a smoking hot body as a senior? -- Cremation.

2. What is a prize old people can win for aging? -- Atrophy.

3. I used to know a couple who grew fruit trees together. They lived to a ripe old age.

4. What's the best part of old age? -- That it doesn't last very long.

5. These are not gray hairs! They are wisdom highlights.

6. Which underwear brand do seniors love best?

It Depends.

7. Old age makes us great multitaskers. Why, I can sneeze and pee at the same time!

8. One benefit of old age is that your secrets are always safe with your friends … because they can't remember them!

9. Age is an issue of mind over matter. If you don't mind getting older, then it really doesn't matter.

10. Why do old people love English muffins so much?

All the nooks and grannies.

11. Stop thinking of them as "hot flashes." Think of them as your inner child playing with matches.

12. How is the moon like dentures? -- Both come out at night.

13. Now that I've gotten older, everything's finally starting to click for me. My knees, my back, my neck …

14. I've decided: Whatever age I am is the new 30!

15. What goes up but never comes down? -- Your age.

16. I called the incontinence hotline recently. They asked if I could hold.

17. You know you're getting old when your birthday cake is a fire hazard.

18. If I ever decide to buy a horse ranch in my old age, I'm going to name it "Pasture Prime."

19. You know you're getting old when your doctor refers you to an archaeologist.

20. You're not getting old; you're becoming a classic.

21. Old age is a heck of a lot better than the alternative.

22. The older we get, the earlier it gets late.

23. You know you're getting old when your birthday cake is a fire hazard.

24. Old people are just young people who have been alive for a very, very long time.

25. With age comes wisdom … and hair in really weird places.

26. Allow me to politely suggest that this be the year you start lying about your age.

27. Don't let aging get you down; it's too hard to get back up again.

28. I'm getting older and wider instead of older and wiser!

29. With old age comes wisdom … and early-bird specials!

30. At my age, the only pole dancing I do is while holding on to the safety bar in the bathtub.

31. When you consider the alternative, old age really isn't so bad.

32. Aging gracefully is a nice way of saying you're slowly looking worse.

(ref: rd.com/article/old-people-jokes)

Most older people don't take offense at jokes like these yet some of the newer generations become enraged and even pass laws to make it illegal to call them by their biological gender.

All of this is no laughing matter. When new generations create laws that force other people to see the world in the way they want to see the world, which is not reality. The idea of a *"hate crime"* which is not the crime itself but rather a determination of what supposedly motivated the crime is foreign to most old people. A crime is an action, not a thought.

Imagine instead of the 32 old people jokes, the list was 32 jokes about women or jokes about some ethnicity or people with a particular disability. Would it be even mildly funny? Would this book have even been allowed to be published? Would the author be guilty of a hate crime?

In case the reader thinks the author is overreacting, note that the U.S. Justice Department has an entire process dedicated to what it determines as hate crimes.

> **The Department of Justice enforces federal hate crimes laws that cover certain crimes committed on the basis of race, color, religion, national origin, sexual orientation, gender, gender identity, or disability. The Department of Justice began prosecuting federal hate crimes cases after the enactment of the Civil Rights Act of 1968.** (ref: justice.gov/hatecrimes/laws-and-policies)

How this relates to old people is that people from previous generations saw crimes as action despite the thoughts behind the action. This is the entire concept of the U.S. judicial system where justice is supposed to be "blind" and not consider supposed motivation for actions. To make a case that a crime was committed because of one of the *Federally protected biases*" forces people to all think the same way. If it is statistically more probable that a blue person will be murdered or raped by a purple person, then when a blue person brandishes a firearm in the company of a hostile purple person, if there is a crime, it should not be considered more forcibly prosecuted because the blue person had a bias against the purple person. We've already seen how raw data is being manipulated to hide the facts.

This is pretty strong stuff for a chapter called Old People Jokes but putting this content here will help drive home the point that adjudicating based on thoughts rather than actions in not funny. It is dangerous and wrong not only in contrast to the U.S. Justice System but to human nature. Maybe this is why the newer generations are trying so hard not to be human anymore.

Notice that among the Federally Protected Biases, age did not make the cut.

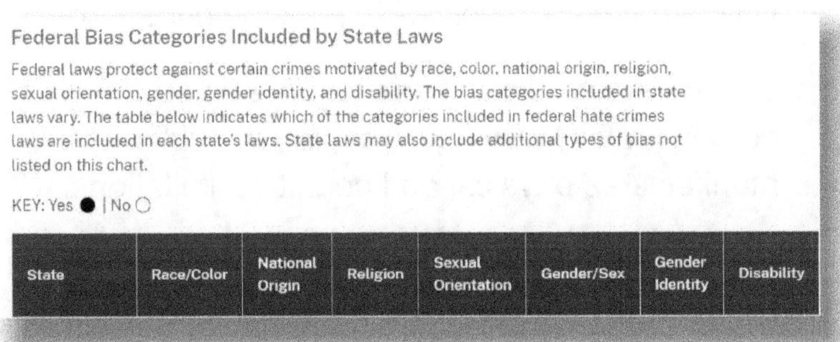

Certainly there are groups that rally against what they label as "*ageism*" which includes a bias against any age of a person, but it is not a covered Federal "hate crime" to randomly punch out and old person walking on the street because you see they are old and most likely can't fight back. It is not a hate crime to rip a purse from an old lady. It is not a hate crime to scope out where old people live so you can break into their houses. It's not a hate crime to target old people with financial frauds because old people tend to be more trusting.

Making these things hate crimes won't correct the inherent issue with classifying anything a hate crime.

Where the law concerns itself most with a person's age is in the area of employment. It is supposed to be illegal to discriminate against a qualified applicant for a job, based solely on the applicant's age.

However, even in politics there is a concern with age.

U.S. president Biden has been observed demonstrating very acute senility in public. This manifests as physical and cognitive limitations.

Just as the U.S. Constitution has a requirement for a minimum age to attain the presidency, perhaps it should consider a maximum age. The inherent "unfairness" in the minimum and maximum is that there are exceptions in both directions where the person operates with a level of maturity, wisdom, and ability.

At the time of this writing the median age of senators in the U.S. Senate was 65.3 years and the oldest being 90.

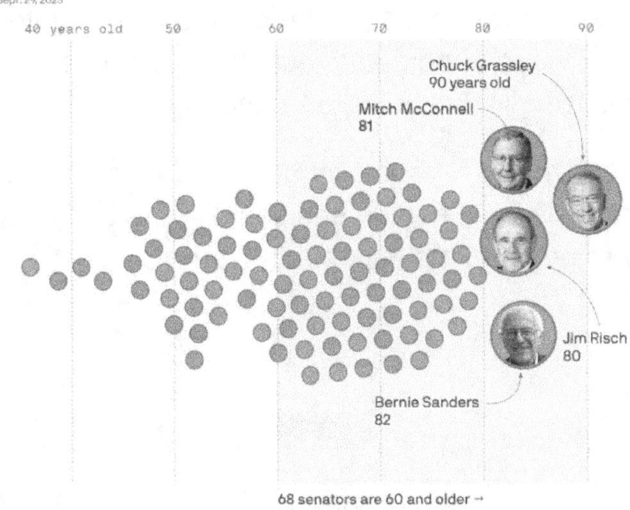

There has been talk of making politicians take cognitive tests after a certain age. Such an idea has also been implied for driver license renewals for the elderly. But how would any of that work without being a contradiction to the entire social justice/equality/equity mantra? Why would it be acceptable to make one group of people pass some qualifier and not other groups where raw data, statistical facts prove out? Suppose black people were not allowed to have jobs in law enforcement because statistically, as we saw from the FBI study, black people are more prone to murder, rape, and theft?

What if left-handed people were denied jobs as truck and bus drivers because the controls are situated for right-handed people and thus there might be a unrealized limitation for left-handed drivers?

As ludicrous as these scenarios might seem, this is exactly how old people see some of the things the newer generations impose on them.

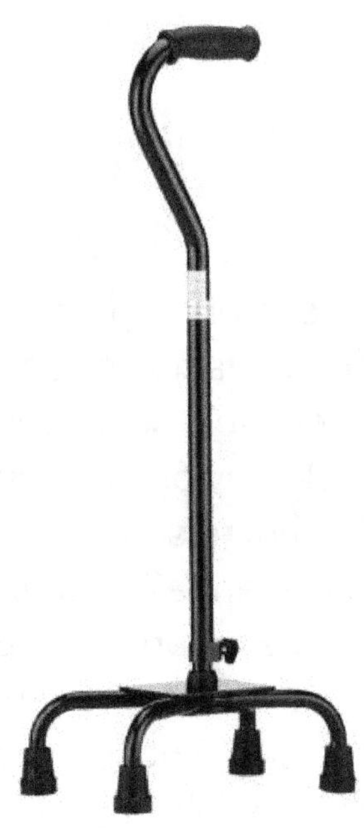

CHAPTER 8 TIMELESSNESS

In every culture there is a deference and honor given to the elderly as wise and experienced. From sentiments like *"respect your elders"* to biblical precepts and warning to not veer from the *"old paths"*, the concept of considering not just old people but also their ideas is repeated all throughout human societies.

With all the discussion about the differences between the previous and current generations, we now move to look for the commonalities. We've already pointed out how this book is not merely about generational differences in slang or preference in music for example. But we're now going to discuss the timeless attributes from generations.

Some of those were already mentioned and have since been abandoned by the newer generations. Many people in the newer generations do not live to work nor do they want to work to live. They seek the bare minimum of interference in their actual living of life. A job is only needed to fund what they really want to be doing. If they can figure out how to fund their life without a typical job, they will.

Some older generations see these younger people as irresponsible leeches and drains waiting for handouts, and yes, some of the people in the newer generations are relying on handouts or even theft to fund their lifestyle. But a larger number of new generation people are developing ways to generate funds in not so typical ways, including social media.

So, we might say one of the timelessness attributes is innovation. Both older and newer generations are the realm of the innovators. Where the previous generations built tangible structures, the architecture of the newer generations is more ethereal and virtual yet just as much a structure.

Previous generations fought physical wars for what they claimed was the advancement of freedom and liberty; allowing people to think and believe as they desire. Newer generations claim they protest and speak out to also advance those same principles even if that freedom allows people to behave or appear odd to other people, specifically the old people.

Unity seemed to be a theme of many older generations. The UNITED states for example over the Confederate states. The United Nations. The European Union. The newer generations also seek unity but seem to be trying to bring it about via social peer pressure. During protests, the newer generations will often chant *"Shame! Shame! Shame!"* in an attempt to shame their opponents to relent.

The newer generations are the generations of "*cancel culture*" and doxxing where enormous, unified efforts are made to publicly force compliance or change.

While their methods seem different than previous generations, perhaps a comparison is how the West has depicted Communism and especially the times during the so-called "*Cold War*" with the former Soviet Union. Some older people in the West have been conditioned to always dislike and distrust Russians.

So the three things we have identified that are common to older and newer generations are:

1. **Innovation**
2. **Freedom**
3. **Unity**

The problem some of the older generations have with the newer generations appeal to these shared principles revolves around perception and morality.

Older generations understood all three of these aspects as being governed by a certain morality.

Morals don't seem to be timeless but rather some morals are contrived with each new generation. What was previously wrong and right may no longer be so.

Without the same moral compass of previous generations, innovation, freedom, and unity take on a different quality not recognized by the older generation.

Innovation and freedom may show itself as more open use of previously profane or social unacceptable behavior such as profanity and public sexual acts.

Unity may manifest as groupthink where any sort of variance to the group is considered discriminatory to the group. The variance is labeled as bigotry and will be mercilessly excoriated into silence or compliance.

Without a moral compass, it is difficult for the previous generations to understand the newer generations. The older generations filter their worldview through concepts of honor, dignity, and self-respect. These things are often foreign to newer generations. They get upset if they have to go to work on their birthday or if someone doesn't call them by their fabricated pronoun.

The timelessness of morality has less to do with religion as some new generations try to dismiss morals and more to do cohesiveness of society.

A society will cease to exist if it doesn't share the same ideas about right and wrong behavior. Perhaps as said, a new type of shared morality is developing among the newer generations. But these morals don't need to be so tightly expressed because of the disconnected nature of the newer generations. A person can live in relative solitude in a world where everything can be accessed online. There is little pressure from the "town" to push for moral compliance.

The very thing that has bound past generations together and made them timeless -- their shared morality – is the very thing that seems to disconnect the newer generations from the previous. While the new generations may have morals, it is difficult to tell what they are.

However, under the surface of the morals of past generations is often a hidden reality. We may have reverence for the grandfatherly old man. We may see him in a light of nostalgic honor. But sometimes there are deep, dark family secrets about our progenitors. The family may know about it but never talks about it. We pretend they are the noble person they project themselves to be. The morals we point out may not be as solid as we think.

The newer generations see no need to keep quiet. They don't want to be keepers of family secrets. They do not feel compelled to honor someone they know is no nobler than they. They do not adhere to the "*don't speak bad things of the dead*". It is a hypocrisy in which they do not want to participate. A hypocrisy that previous generations maintained as part of being "*civil*". Whether the hypocrisy is in your own family or is of a president that took showers with his teenage daughter and caused so much trauma that she wrote about it in her diary. (ref: wtrf.com/top-stories/alleged-showers-with-my-dad-president-joe-bidens-daughter-reportedly-writes-of-abuse-in-diary)

The point is not to make this political but to show that this hypocrisy isn't something relegated to the "*common people*" but happens at all social strata.

The timelessness may not be the three things listed but more that humans are humans; flawed creatures that often pretend to be better and more civilized than they are.

Each generation needs to seek the "glue" that holds society together. That holds the past to the present and the future.

The hypocrisy goes both ways. The newer generations often rally for causes like ending petroleum-based products including oil and gasoline as a way to "save the planet" but at the same time, these newer generations must have their clothing and devices often made from the same resources they are trying to end. Further, the hypocrisy comes when the newer generations behave like everything is so dire but they live fairly pampered lives.

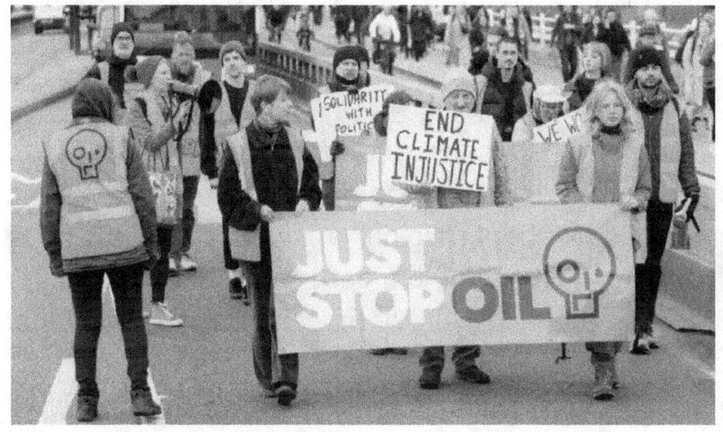

There are those moments when the previous and newer generations coalesce and begin to understand their differences and similarities. When the racist old man holds his half-black grandchild and forgets he was ever a racist. When the pierced and tattooed Gen-Zer has that ah-ha moment that those wartime video games he is playing are based on the actual times their grandfather or great-grandfather lived.

An older person might see in a younger, their own rebellious youth stage. The younger person may see in the older, their future self. But as the generations become less similar, the disconnect becomes more stark.

Finally, when speaking of timelessness and how morals are the heart of the generational connection, we must talk about religion. Not just Christianity as is dominant in the West, but generically all religions. Religions are the basis for most moral systems. Or at least religions act as the conduits to convey societal morality. So, the further away people move from their society's dominant religion, the least likely they will share the same morals as previous generations.

As newer generations question the legitimacy not only of religion but the morals that accompany those religions, they become unmoored from the "glue" that holds together the society in which they were raised. In this disconnected state, they are willing to accept almost anything since they have not settled on a new moral system. Any principles they may exhibit are fluid, inconsistent, and even hypocritical. To make matters worse, most religions are based on repeated experiences of a society. For example, while there may be a story of how a deity imposed which day is the prime day to worship, stripping away that supernatural possibility, a society will have learned from experience that the population needs a time when the entire community focuses on their shared morality; to reinforce those morals and bolster the unity of the society.

The erosion of a society's shared morals will dismantle the society and allow it to be replaced. The timelessness comes to an end.

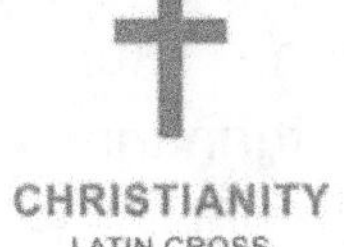

CHRISTIANITY
LATIN CROSS

ISLAM
CRESCENT AND STAR

HINDUISM
AUM LETTER

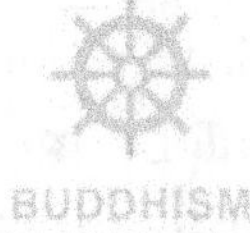

BUDDHISM
DHARMACHAKRA

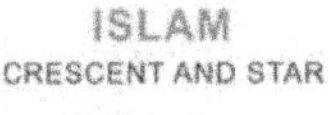

TAOISM
YIN AND YANG

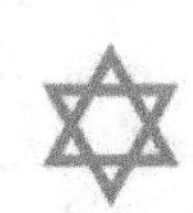

SHINTO
TORII GATE

JUDAISM
STAR OF DAVID

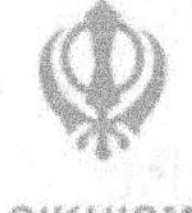

SIKHISM
KHANDA

CHAPTER 9 AFTER YOU

Old people of every generation eventually realize their time is coming to an end. Their influence is waning. Their stars are fading. They will sometimes complain how time is passing them by and how processes and technology have become too complex for them. They may joke about how they have become their fathers. Such sentiment is captured in the song by Harry Chapin, *Cat's in the Cradle* (ref: youtu.be/KUwjNBjqR-c) where the lyrics recount a son that constantly seeks the attention of his dad but the dad never seems to have time. The child idolizes the dad nonetheless and wants to grow up to be just like his dad. Eventually, the adult child does grow up and has no time for his elderly father.

But the world will not stop once you are gone. There will be multiple more generations stranger than the one you rail against the most. There will be new processes, new technologies, and new morality systems. Well, unless the apocalyptic stories of many of the religions are true, then it might all cease to exist.

Just like your father and grandfather, you'll be amazed and sometimes disgusted at the new things you see.

However, fret not. Your generation has left a mark on the world; good and bad. Future generations will both benefit from and have to clean up messes your generation passed on. There is no golden generation. Each one has its flaws. No matter how "*cool*" or advanced any generation may think of themselves, they too will be eclipsed by future generations.

The danger in the author's present time is that many in the subsequent generations do not want to fulfill roles that are essential for the continuance of civilization. Many no longer want to be police officers or paramedics or "*first responders*" of any kind. There seems to be less desire and incentive to be something special. The days of the innovators may be gone. We may be at the Destroyer stage of the generational cycle.

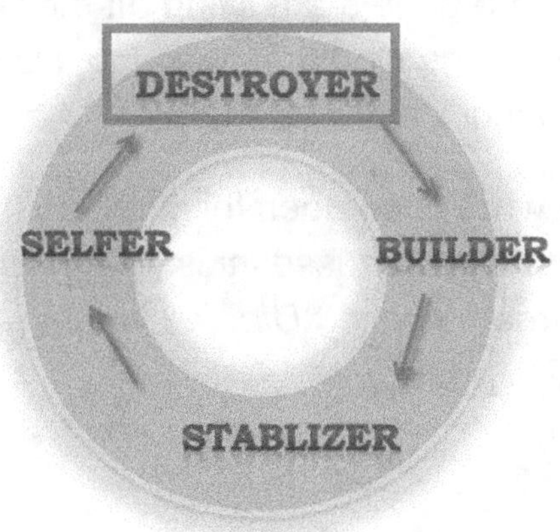

In any science fiction scenario where someone from the past is brought into the future, the experience is both wondrous and frightening to the person. Imagine yourself being brought back from the dead into a world where the distinctions between male and female are not apparent. A future where humans are augmented with cybernetic implants instead of holding cell phones in their hands. A time when there are no borders and no nations but rather the world is one giant, sprawling city with industrial, commercial, and environmental zones. Perhaps there will be complete automation as envisioned by the author in one of his articles. (ref: rodericke.com/ff) Where no one works because machines do it all including repairing themselves. There are no classes because the financial divide is gone since currency and the need for currency has been eliminated. People are free to pursue their passions instead of working their entire lives to pay bills. There would be no complaint about how some people are living off the labor of others since no one would be working. No more taxes to collect. No more embezzlement.

However, at what price does this utopian future come? The author discusses this in a 9 minute "movie" he created called *Utopia Undone*. (ref: youtu.be/8JZ5DSQDrwU)

Along with all the exciting benefits of the future imagined by the author could come the unimaginable limitations. Perhaps self-driving electric automobiles replace any ability for a person to sit behind the wheel of an internal combustion, gas guzzling 57 Chevy.

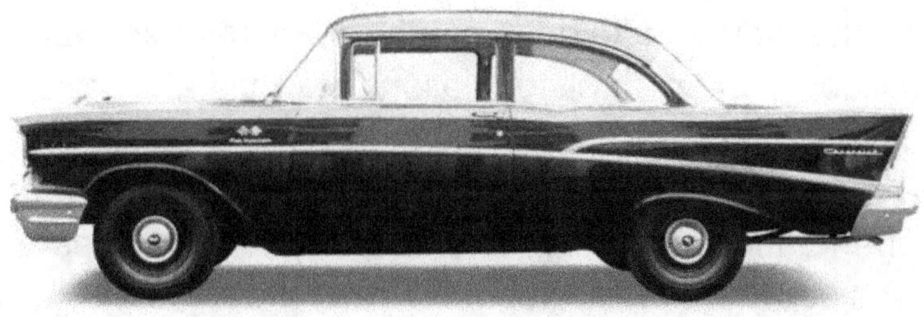

There may be a limit to how much food you can have. A limit on the size of the dwelling where you live. Already, in the author's time there is a push to create what are called 15-Minute cities.

The 15-Minute City concept is supposed to address what is called "sprawl", where people move away from population centers and by so doing not only encroach upon former wilderness spaces but also take commerce away from the cities, thus often leaving the cities impoverished and vacant.

The 15-Minute City "*is an urban planning concept in which most daily necessities and services, such as work, shopping, education, healthcare, and leisure can be easily reached by a 15-minute walk, bike ride, or public transit ride from any point in the city.*" (ref: en.wikipedia.org/wiki/15-minute_city)

While some people may welcome the concept, it has its detractors that worry that constraining populations like this would invite governments to more effectively lockdown and control populations. It would allow the implementation of many programs which are difficult to do when people live on the outskirts or so-called "off-the-grid" where they rely little on public services such as water and sewage.

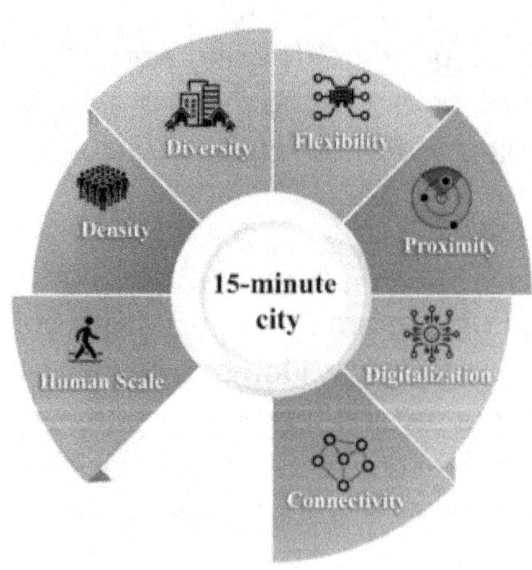

Another effort to radically alter the future is in the area of DNA manipulation. Some of it comes in the form of GMOs or genetically modified organisms in food such as adding modified bacteria DNA to reduce attacks by insects or pro-long the shelf-life of produce. Another form of DNA manipulation is used to attempt cross-species breeding such as half-human half-animal "chimeras". While, so far the scientists performing these half-breeds supposedly terminate after the embryo stage, citing ethics there will come a time when they allow the experiment to go to term. You could see a half-human half-ape in your future and perhaps live your own version of the movie series, *Planet of the Apes*.

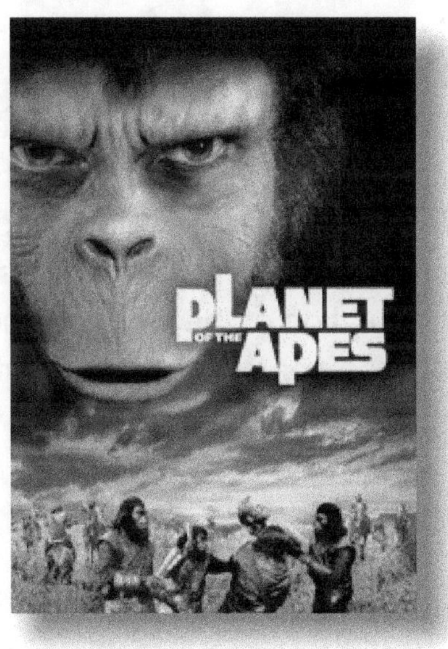

But perhaps the most sinister use of DNA manipulation is in the form of altering "vaccines" for human use. Previously, vaccines were created from cultures, sometimes even from the dormant virus being combated. However, by the time the Covid-19 virus struck the entire planet, pharmaceutical companies were using mRNA vaccines which alters genes to create or "message" an immune response. (ref: en.wikipedia.org/wiki/MRNA_vaccine)

Not everyone is as positive with the use of mRNA vaccines as some people cite the "died suddenly" syndrome effects where more young people appear to be dying suddenly without any prior health warning, often from heart conditions not typically seen in youth.

In fact, a 2022 documentary film called *Died Suddenly* was produced that alleges that the Covid-19 vaccine is being used as a concerted effort at depopulation. (ref: diedsuddenly.info/) While this claim has been dismissed by the "experts" as a wild conspiracy theory, there are verified and public efforts to decrease the population of the world, sometimes by half; by over 4 billion people. How can that be done but by some massive program?

To make this point, the author cites these quotes by influential people that are on record advocating decreasing the world population by significant amounts.

"First, we've got population. The world today has 6.8 billion people. That's headed up to about nine billion. Now, if we do a really great job on new vaccines, health care, reproductive health services, we could lower that by, perhaps, 10 or 15 percent. But there, we see an increase of about 1.3." – Bill Gates (ref: ted.com/talks/bill_gates_innovating_to_zer o/transcript)

"Overpopulation in various countries has become a serious threat to the well-being of many people and a grave obstacle to any attempt to organize peace on this planet of ours." – Albert Einstein (ref: populationmatters.org/quotes)

> **"In the last 200 years the population of our planet has grown exponentially, at a rate of 1.9 per cent per year. If it continued at this rate, with the population doubling every 40 years, by 2600 we would all be standing literally shoulder to shoulder."** – Stephen Hawking (ref: populationmatters.org/quotes)

There is even a program by the United Nations, under the guise of "sustainability" to depopulate the world. This program is called *Agenda 21* (ref: sdgs.un.org/publications/agenda21)

Some people cite this UN program as a nefarious attempt to "sustain" the population. But like in the case of responses to so many globalized programs, people who oppose mRNA programs or UN depopulation programs disguised as environmental programs are dismissed as *"right-wing conspiracy theorists"*.

So, whether the future is bright or bleak, it seems for it to move forward will require that all old people, old ways, old thinking, must die, through direct depopulation or generational attrition.

Chapter 10 Conclusion

Speaking of dismissals, some people that consume this book will dismiss it as the ramblings of a "riiiiiight-wing extremist" no matter how many reference links are provided. The sources will be dismissed as merely easy to edit open-source Wikipedia fare or cherry-picked "conservative propaganda click-bait" even though Wikipedia is dominated by collectivists and most of the references were of the actual advocates or documents of the topic discussed.

But this book and this author is not trying to present one side of anything. The attempt is to write to the future before narrative and real propaganda all but silences any other voice no matter how prolific the sourced evidence. Even the evidence will be erased, leaving the consumer of material like this believing the claims that it is merely the rantings of a madman.

We set out with an alarming title. ***All Old People Must Die***. The title encapsulates not just the expiry of physically old people and how it is simply an inevitability that their kind are being replaced every day, but how old ideas and old worldviews are being replaced.

But this book, like all RoderickE books wasn't meant to be a book you read and put back on the shelf. These books peer into the past, present, and future to glean out of time and space, the reality of the topics.

These books are not trendy or placating to any one philosophy. RoderickE books get just as many negative reviews as they do positive. This kind of content isn't warm and fuzzy. It is mind-changing or at least thought provoking.

How has this content affected you? Are you an "old" person that picked up this book because of the title? Are you a young person given this book by a friend that insisted you read it?

Old people contribute more to the lives of younger people than they might realize. Besides the wisdom and experience of their lives, older people pass on basic knowledge of skills not taught in schools. There is a reason many of the architecture and automobile designs of today are bland edges and rectangles rather than the smooth curves and detailed craftsmanship of times past. There is no desire to expend all the time and effort to do anything beyond the utilitarian purpose. Why add pointless flared wheel wells to a car? Why make domed rotundas in buildings? Even dining rooms and hallways are wasted spaces in houses.

This is not to say that the newer generations aren't creative but their attention to the details as the older generations is different.

However, if the newer generations continue to be disinterested in bridge-building, in gears and pulleys, in farming, in animal husbandry, in woodworking and masonry – eventually there will be no "old people" left to show them the tricks of those trades not recorded in books or clickable on a YouTube video. Entire trades could be lost.

Maybe it won't matter. Maybe these are the death throes, the last gasps of a Luddite generation kicking and screaming to stay in the past. The cotton gin is gone. No one turns its crank. The victrola either, let alone pushing the next track on an 8-track player.

While nostalgic, those things have no place in this world anymore. Even the most recent gizmo of today will be replaced tomorrow. Some of it is even planned, such as in the concept of *planned obsolescence* wherein products are designed to fail after a certain time so that the consumer will buy the replacement.

It seems whether by evolution or deity, the human race is operating under a sort of planned obsolescence. The older generation cannot remain forever even through gene manipulation or cryo-freezers.

The old people must die. They must make way for the next best thing… or worst thing that will replace them.

But fortunately we have writing. We have audio and video. We have digital record of many things. It will not take some accidental discovery to look very far back and see what we were. Who we were.

We must not ponder too long. Think too long. The future awaits!

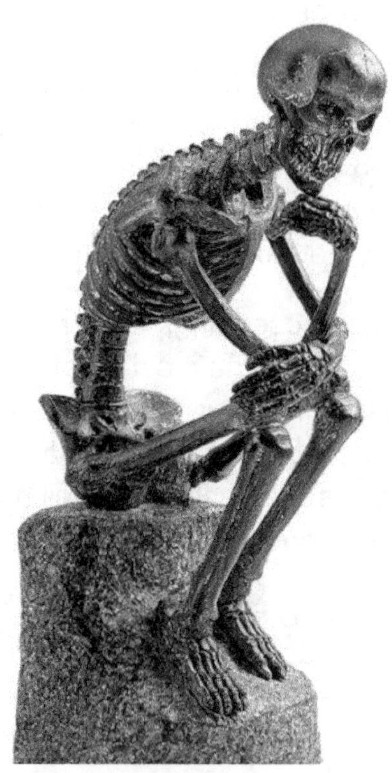

Would you be interested in joining or starting a book group to discuss the topics discussed in this book?

To contact Roderick Edwards, go to rodericke.com/contact and send an email directly to him. Not to an agent or staff.

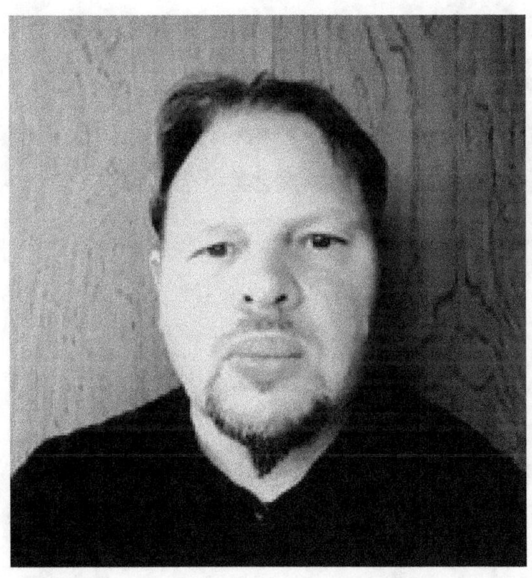

About The Author

RODERICK EDWARDS is a multi-genre author that was adopted at age 4 and found his birth family at age 50. A lifetime of being an outsider has afforded him the unique opportunity to see human behavior as if he were examining it from another planet.

Whether he is writing a Microsoft Excel help book or an autobiography or a fictional tale of a person on a deserted planet, all of his books come with this special perspective that cannot be duplicated by another author.

Every person that reads a Roderick Edwards book is treated to an almost personal one-on-one conversation with Roderick.

Find out more at
amazon.com/author/roderickedwards

Or visit rodericke.com

OTHER BOOKS BY RODERICK

rodericke.com

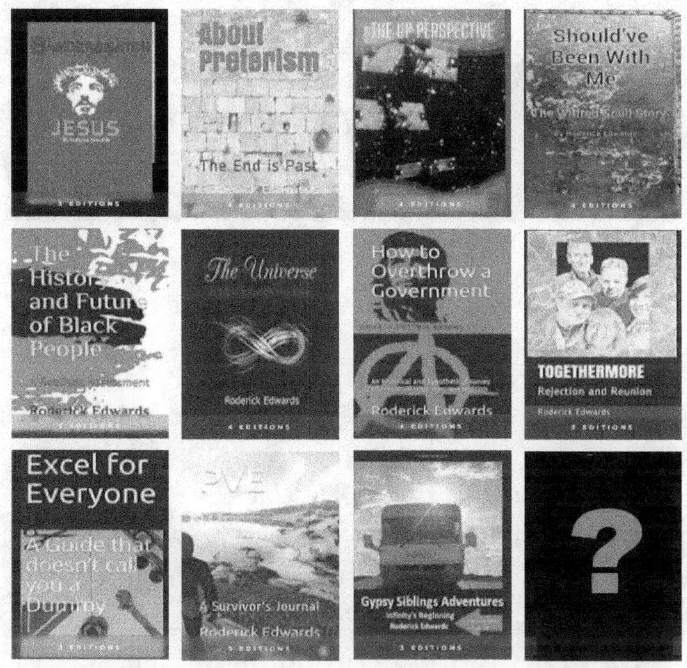

SEE ALSO, many of these titles are available as AUDIOBOOKS!!!

audible.com/author/B07B9R59Q2

WHAT NEXT?

Now that you've read this book, what's next? Why not try another RoderickE book. RoderickE is a multi-genre author. Select a genre you like best.

- https://rodericke.com/FICTION
- https://rodericke.com/NONFICTION
- https://rodericke.com/POLITICS
- https://rodericke.com/RELIGION
- https://rodericke.com/HISTORY
- https://rodericke.com/PHILOSOPHY
- https://rodericke.com/TECHNICAL
- https://rodericke.com/CULTURE
- https://rodericke.com/OTHER

www.ingramcontent.com/pod-product-compliance
Lightning Source LLC
Chambersburg PA
CBHW060748260726
48660CB00002B/532